Blood Pressure;

Lower Your Blood Pressure Today with Delicious Foods, 20 Recipes Fighting High Blood Pressure and Win with Healthy Natural Foods

by M Laurence

Table of Contents

1. Introduction to High Blood Pressure

High Blood Pressure is often referred to as a 'silent killer' - You can't see it, or smell it and sometimes the symptoms can be hard to impossible to detect. In fact you can think you are perfectly healthy until you get a checkup at the Doctor and are told your blood pressure is too high. This of course can be like a bombshell especially if you feel are healthy. Worse while you take in that alarming information you are prescribed a cocktail of drugs. And so before you now it you're taking regular pills day after day, week after week, and worse year after year.

While drugs are a good option to immediately lower particularly high blood pressure, they come with a host of side effects. Even if they don't come with side-effects the thought of taking drugs for what could be years is not appealing.

High blood pressure causes at least 7.6 million premature deaths worldwide. In the UK alone every day there are 350 preventable strokes or heart attacks due to high blood pressure. Approximately 16 million people in the UK have high blood pressure, including a third who do not even know they have it.

What Exactly is Blood Pressure?

Blood pressure is measured in millimetres of mercury (mmHg) and is recorded as two figures:

- systolic pressure – the pressure of the blood when your heart beats to pump blood out
- diastolic pressure – the pressure of the blood when your heart rests in between beats, which reflects how strongly your arteries are resisting blood flow

For example if your Doctor/GP says your blood pressure is "120 over 80", or 120/80mmHg, it means you have a systolic pressure of 120mmHg and a diastolic pressure of 80mmHg.

So now we know what it means - what should our pressure actually be? Ideally, we should all have a blood pressure below 120 over 80 (120/80). If your blood pressure is above 120/80 you will need to lower it.

Most adults in the UK/US have blood pressure readings in the range from 120 over 80 (120/80) to 140 over 90 (140/90). If your blood pressure is within this range then you should be taking steps to bring it down or to stop it rising any further at the very least.

The higher your blood pressure, the higher your risk of health problems. For example, someone with a blood pressure level of 135 over 85 (135/85) is twice as likely to have a heart attack or stroke as someone with a reading of 115 over 75 (115/75).

The Dangers of High Blood Pressure

High blood pressure (hypertension) puts extra strain on your heart and blood vessels. This can cause them to become damaged or weakened.

High blood pressure can affect your body in a number of ways:

- Your heart: high blood pressure can cause you to have a heart attack. It can also cause heart failure.
- Your brain: high blood pressure is a leading cause of strokes. It has also been closely linked to some forms of dementia.
- Your kidneys: high blood pressure can cause kidney disease.
- Your limbs: high blood pressure can cause peripheral arterial disease, which can affect your legs.

Side-Effects

Once diagnosed with high blood pressure the unusual route is to see a Doctor who prescribes you medication to potentially take for the rest of your life. Not only that these drugs can have a variety of side-effects from:

- Feeling drowsy.
- Pain around your kidney area (on the side of your lower back)
- A dry cough.

- Dizziness, faintness or light headedness.
- Skin rash.
- Swelling of your feet.

As I said while I do agree medication can reduce your blood pressure fast, which is great for a short term solution, you may want something else long term. Something natural to work alongside the medication and eventually get rid of the drugs and pills. That's where this book comes in with an armoury of different foods and strategies to combat high blood pressure - the natural way.

What can we do to fight Blood Pressure Naturally?

There are a number of things - but your diet is number one - what you eat and drink has a real effect on your heart and blood pressure. If you have high blood pressure, it is even more important to make healthy changes to your diet.

For a few people, following blood pressure friendly eating habits may help them to avoid medicines altogether. Yes - getting you completely off of those tablets and back to living a normal drug-free life without the horrible side-effects.

Research now shows that it's just as important to choose foods naturally low in sodium and high in at least two of the three power minerals: calcium, magnesium, and potassium.

Which foods are these? What can we do with these foods to make them easily edible for daily life? Intrigued? Let us work together and lower your blood pressure - for good!

2. Just Why is High Salt Intake so Bad?

One of the quickest ways to lower your blood pressure (especially if you have particularly high blood pressure) is to eat less salt.

Why salt is bad

Everyone prattles on about salt being bad, but why exactly is it bad? After a fast food burger and chips have you ever feel bloated later on in the evening? Have you needed a sit down after that huge pizza and soft drink? Or after a curry and beer ever had a poor night's sleep and got up to get water?

If yes that's because fast food is loaded with salt and salt makes your body retain water. If you eat too much, the extra water stored in your body raises your blood pressure. This can be a particular problem if you already have high blood pressure.

On a side note eating too much salt may mean that blood pressure medicines you are already taking including diuretics, won't work as well.

The higher your blood pressure, the greater the strain all this retained water will put on your heart, arteries, kidneys and brain. This can lead to heart attacks, strokes, and dementia and kidney disease.

How much salt is too much?

An adult should eat no more than 6g of salt a day, but most of us eat much more than this.

Most of the salt we eat every day is "hidden". Did you know that roughly 80% of the salt we eat is hiding in processed foods?

Food like:

- bacon, ham and smoked meats
- cheese
- pickles
- salami
- salted and dry roasted nuts
- salt fish and smoked fish
- soy sauce
- gravy granules, stock cubes and yeast extract
- bread
- biscuits
- breakfast cereals
- prepared ready meals
- takeaways

Incredibly only 20% comes from the salt we add while cooking or at the table. That's means we are only controlling 1/5th of our own salt intake! So we must be more vigilant about what we put inside our body.

What salt levels mean

To avoid the hidden salt and cut down your salt intake, it is best to eat foods that are low in salt and stop using salt when cooking or at the table.

Firstly take your control back. Get used to reading labels and what to look for:

- Low - 0.3g salt or less per 100g of food - Eat plenty of these
- Medium - 0.3-1.5g salt per 100g of food - Eat small amounts occasionally
- High - 1.5g salt or more per 100g of food - Avoid these completely

What sodium levels mean

Some labels may not say how much salt the food contains, but may say how much sodium it contains. Sodium is one of the chemicals in salt. 1g of sodium is the same as 2.5g of salt.

- Low - 0.1g sodium or less per 100g of food - Eat plenty of these
- Medium - 0.1-0.6g sodium per 100g of food - Eat small amounts occasionally
- High - 0.6 sodium or more per 100g of food - Avoid if possible

It's another way of confusing the consumer whether something is low in Salt or Sodium. So try to reduce your Salt intake and be aware of labels. This can hugely help your Blood Pressure and reduce bloating and water retention.

3. Great Ways to Eat Less Salt

I wanted to create a list of quick reference solutions to avoid and lower Salt - here are some great ideas:

1. Try out different herbs and spices - and from seasonings like chili, ginger, lime or lemon juice.
2. Avoid adding salt when cooking also this includes things like soy sauce, curry powders and stock cubes.
3. If you really can't do without a salty favour, you could try using a small amount of low-sodium salt substitute. If you have kidney problems or diabetes, check with your doctor or nurse first.
4. There are a number of table sauces now that specifically sell 'low salt' options and still taste great. Sauces like ketchup, brown sauce, mustard and pickles can contain a lot of salt. Check the label and choose low-salt options.
5. Bread and breakfast cereals can contain a lot of salt. Check the labels to compare brands. Can you change to something like porridge? Muesli? Scrambled Egg? Something less manufactured and more natural.
6. Smoked meats and some tinned fish contain a lot of salt. Avoid these if you can.
7. If you are eating out, ask if your meal can be made with less salt. This obviously may not be possible and also you don't eat out a lot then i personally wouldn't bother. When you start depriving yourself of a meal with friends you'll resent you new diet. Don't deprive yourself of enjoying a meal out. If you eat out regularly then this is something to certainly look at.

8. Get to know low-salt recipes. Enjoy the process of looking for tasty alternatives. There are a number of low-salt cookbooks available - of which i am working on.
9. Don't be too fussed about the exact amount of salt you eat. Try to always eat foods with the lowest salt level. 6g of salt a day is the maximum you should eat, and the less you eat the better.

A final note would be don't turn food into a chore. Aim for eating healthy for 3 days out of 4 for 2 weeks then slowly work up to 6 days out of 7. So when you go out with friends for a meal you're not eating just a salad while everyone enjoys a burger. Crucially it's YOU who wants to change and make a difference to your long term heath. You can do this - but baby steps first. Reduce Salt and Sodium. Second introduce foods that specifically are good at lowering blood pressure which I'm going to cover next.

4. Dark Chocolate Tarts

According to a study published in the Journal of the American Medical Association eating about 30 calories a day of dark chocolate - just one tiny square - was shown to help lower blood pressure after 18 weeks without weight gain or other adverse effects. So this is a great way to lower your blood pressure right off the bat.

The compounds in dark chocolate appear to be highly protective against the oxidation of LDL. In the long term, this should cause much less cholesterol to lodge in the arteries and we should see a lower risk of heart disease over the long term.

Another study showed that eating dark chocolate 5 plus times per week lowered the risk of cardiovascular disease by 57% - this again was in small bite sized chunks.

Choose dark chocolate consisting of at least 70 percent cocoa powder. Because chocolate is typically high in calories, be careful how much you consume. 1 to 2 squares a day is perfectly fine.

Dark Chocolate Tarts

Ingredients

- plain flour, for dusting
- 375g/13oz ready-made shortcrust pastry
- 250g/8oz dark chocolate, roughly chopped
- 250ml/8floz double cream
- 75g/3oz stem ginger, finely chopped

This is a great little cheat if you want to do something more interesting that just eating a square of dark chocolate a day.

Preheat the oven to 200C/400F/Gas 6.

Dust the work surface with flour and roll the ready-made dough out thinly. Use it to line one large 25cm/10in tart ring or 6 individual tartlet rings 10cm/4in in diameter. Then once done just trim away any excess.

Line the tart case with baking parchment, fill with baking beans and bake in the oven for around 12-15 minutes.

Remove the baking beans and paper and then cook for a further 10 minutes or until the base of the tart is golden-brown and cooked through. Then remove the tart from the oven and set aside to cool.

Meanwhile, if you heat the chocolate and cream in a saucepan set over a medium heat, stirring continuously until the chocolate melts and mixture is smooth and thick. This should smell fantastic.

Sprinkle the finely chopped stem ginger over the base of the tart, reserving a little to garnish.

Pour the chocolate mixture into the tart shell and then leave to chill in the fridge for 45 minutes. This maybe a touch longer but you want the chococate to set. Sprinkle over the remaining stem ginger and enjoy!

Nutrition Facts - Dark Chocolate

A 100 gram bar of dark chocolate with 70-85% cocoa contains

Amount Per 100 grams	
Calories	546
% Daily Value*	
Total Fat 31 g	47%
Saturated fat 19 g	95%
Polyunsaturated fat 1.1 g	
Monounsaturated fat 10 g	
Trans fat 0.1 g	
Cholesterol 8 mg	2%
Sodium 24 mg	1%
Potassium 559 mg	15%
Total Carbohydrate 61 g	20%
Dietary fiber 7 g	28%
Sugar 48 g	
Protein 4.9 g	9%
Caffeine 43 mg	
Vitamin A	1%
Vitamin C	0%
Calcium	5%
Iron	67%
Vitamin D	0%

Vitamin B-6	0%
Vitamin B-12	3%
Magnesium	58%

5. Beetroot Smoothie

Beetroot has been gaining some ground recently as a super food. In 2010 UK researchers revealed a nitrate which is the special ingredient in beetroot can lower blood pressure and may help to fight heart disease. When ingested, scientists believe our body converts nitrates into nitric oxide, a chemical thought to lower blood pressure.

Drinking beetroot juice increases blood flow to the brain in older people, which may be able to fight the progression of dementia, a 2010 study suggested.

Of course you can buy Beetroots in jars and these are great for adding to a salad if you're short of time. You can buy raw Beetroots in any food super store and a great way to eat them is to make a smoothie. Add two Beetroots, two apples, some ginger and ice to a blender. Thats a potent drink for combating high blood pressure.

Beetroot Smoothie

Ingredients

- 2 Raw Beetroot
- 1 apple
- handful of blueberries
- tiny slice ginger to create a smooth and nutritious drink with depth and zing.
- Ice to thicken and cool

Mix all these together in a blender. You can experiment with more or less ginger depending on flavour.

Nutrition Facts - Beetroot

Beetroot

Amount Per 100 grams

Calories	43
% Daily Value*	
Total Fat 0.2 g	0%
Saturated fat 0 g	0%
Polyunsaturated fat 0.1 g	
Monounsaturated fat 0 g	
Cholesterol 0 mg	0%
Sodium 78 mg	3%
Potassium 325 mg	9%
Total Carbohydrate 10 g	3%
Dietary fiber 2.8 g	11%
Sugar 7 g	
Protein 1.6 g	3%
Vitamin A	0%
Vitamin C	8%
Calcium	1%
Iron	4%
Vitamin D	0%
Vitamin B-6	5%
Vitamin B-12	0%
Magnesium	5%

6. Greek Yogurt Pancakes

Greek yogurt not only tastes great and makes a healthy dessert it also has some potent nutrients. One cup of fat-free plain yogurt provides 49% of the calcium, 12% of the magnesium, and 18% of the potassium you need every day.

The American Heart Association's High Blood Pressure Research in 2012 found that long-term yogurt eaters had a lower systolic blood pressure, as well as a diminished risk of developing high blood pressure.

Greek yogurt is great with a multitude of foods - how about breakfast with granola? A favorite on it's own or adding fruit. to create more flavour.

Ingredients

- One 5.3-ounce container nonfat Greek Yogurt (any flavor- see *Tips)
- 1 large egg (or 2 large egg whites)
- 1/2 cup Gold Medal® All-Purpose Flour
- 1 teaspoon baking soda
- 1/2 cup fresh blueberries (or 1/2 large banana)

Mix the Greek yogurt and 1 large egg in a medium bowl and blend until smooth. Add flour and baking soda and stir until the dry ingredients are mixed in. The batter will be nice and thick.

Preheat a large pan to medium heat and spray with nonstick spray. Now for the fun part. Use an ice cream scoop or 1/4 to 1/3 cup measuring cup to scoop the batter into the pan. Spread each of the batter scoops into an even circle. Add blueberries or bananas on top of each pancake.

Then cook for about 3 minutes or until nice and golden, then flip and cook the other side for about 2 minutes, until it is golden too. Then just repeat with the remaining batter.

You can serve with additional fruit or just go for honey or syrup.

Nutrition Facts - Greek Yogurt

Yogurt - Greek - nonfat

Amount Per 100 grams

Calories	59

% Daily Value*	
Total Fat 0.4 g	0%
Saturated fat 0.1 g	0%
Polyunsaturated fat 0 g	
Monounsaturated fat 0.1 g	
Trans fat 0 g	

Cholesterol 5 mg	1%
Sodium 36 mg	1%
Potassium 141 mg	4%
Total Carbohydrate 3.6 g	1%
Dietary fiber 0 g	0%
Sugar 3.2 g	
Protein 10 g	20%
Vitamin A	0%
Vitamin C	0%
Calcium	11%
Iron	0%
Vitamin D	0%
Vitamin B-6	5%
Vitamin B-12	13%
Magnesium	2%

7. Peach Crumble in a Mug

Peaches are rich in many vital minerals including potassium, fluoride and iron. Iron is required for red blood cell formation. Potassium is an important component of cell and body fluids that help regulate heart rate and blood pressure. Fluoride is a component of bones and teeth and is essential for prevention of dental caries.

One medium peach or nectarine provides 1% of the calcium, 3% of the magnesium, and 8% of the potassium you need every day.

Not terribly high in Vitamin C but a great fruit to eat on the go.

Peaches Crumble

Ingredients

- 2 tbsp quick oats
- 1 tbsp flour
- 2 tsp butter
- 3 tsp brown sugar
- A pinch cinnamon
- A pinch salt
- 2 peaches, peeled and chopped
- 1/2 tsp lemon juice
- Pinch lemon zest

So firstly you stir oats with flour, butter, 1 tsp brown sugar, cinnamon and salt in a small frying pan over medium high. Make sure it's all mixed well and cook until mixture is crumbly. Make sure it becomes golden, the flour is cooked through. It'll take around 3 to 5 min.

Then add the peaches with 2 tsp brown sugar, lemon juice and zest in a mug. Place in a microwave on high for 1 minute.

Place the crumble over peaches and serve with ice cream!

Nutrition Facts - Peach

Peaches

Amount Per 100 grams

Calories	39

% Daily Value*	
Total Fat 0.2 g	0%
Saturated fat 0 g	0%
Polyunsaturated fat 0.1 g	
Monounsaturated fat 0.1 g	
Cholesterol 0 mg	0%
Sodium 0 mg	0%
Potassium 190 mg	5%
Total Carbohydrate 10 g	3%
Dietary fiber 1.5 g	6%
Sugar 8 g	
Protein 0.9 g	1%

Vitamin A	6%
Vitamin C	11%
Calcium	0%
Iron	1%
Vitamin D	0%
Vitamin B-6	0%
Vitamin B-12	0%
Magnesium	2%

8. Broccoli Smoothie - with Blueberries

Broccoli is a true superfood and just one cup of cooked broccoli provides 6% of the calcium, 8% of the magnesium, and 14% of the potassium you need every day.

A small study from 2012 conducted on 81 people with diabetes, found that those in a group that ate 10g a day of enriched broccoli sprouts powder for four weeks saw a reduction in their levels of cholesterol and triglycerides - both of which can cause cardiovascular disease.

This cruciferous veggie is also a famous source of cancer-fighting phytonutrients called glucosinolates. Have a look at this super powered smoothie.

Brocolli and Blueberries Smoothie

Ingredients

- 1 Cup Water
- 1 Cup Dairy Free Milk
- 1 Cup Blueberries
- 1 Banana
- 1 Cup Broccoli
- 1 Cup Oats (use raw oat groats if following a raw food diet) (Like this)
- 2 Tablespoons Sunflower Seeds (Like this)
- ½ Cup Raisins (or any other dried fruit)

Blend the dry ingredients first - Oats, Raisins, Sunflower seeds, and liquid first for a short time. Empty to a separate container.

Blend the greens - Broccoli next for a short time. Make sure it's fully blended.

Then add the fruit and the rest of the ingredients until smooth and add the dry ingredients next - Oats etc too and mix thoroughly.

If the smoothie is a little too thick add water and to give a cooler taste add a handful of ice - enjoy!

Nutrition Facts - Broccoli

Broccoli

Amount Per 100 grams

Calories	34

% Daily Value*	
Total Fat 0.4 g	0%
Saturated fat 0 g	0%
Polyunsaturated fat 0 g	
Monounsaturated fat 0 g	
Cholesterol 0 mg	0%
Sodium 33 mg	1%
Potassium 316 mg	9%
Total Carbohydrate 7 g	2%

Dietary fiber 2.6 g	10%
Sugar 1.7 g	
Protein 2.8 g	5%
Vitamin A	12%
Vitamin C	148%
Calcium	4%
Iron	3%
Vitamin D	0%
Vitamin B-6	10%
Vitamin B-12	0%
Magnesium	5%

9. Curried Adzuki Beans

Adzuki beans (including black, white, navy, lima, pinto, and kidney) are not only incredibly tasty but are chock-full of soluble fiber, magnesium, and potassium - all excellent ingredients for lowering blood pressure and improving overall heart health. Potassium relaxes blood vessels and increases blood flow, thereby reducing blood pressure and strain on the heart.

Adzuki beans (and the others) are high in dietary fiber which is a key element of digestive health. Fiber also helps to eliminate constipation, diarrhea, and bloating, as well as more serious conditions like colon cancer. So these are great to help with any problems with going to the loo.

Adzuki beans contain a unique mineral known as molybdenum which plays a crucial part in the detoxification of the liver. Even a half-serving of Adzuki beans provides 100% of the daily recommended intake.

Here's a tasty one-dish meal that's high in calcium and spices to boost circulation. Small, reddish-brown adzuki beans have a sweet flavor. They have a higher protein content than other beans and are easier to digest.

Curried Beans - serves 6

Ingredients

- 1 cup adzuki beans, picked over and rinsed
- 1 Tbs. olive oil
- ½ cup diced yellow onion
- 2 cloves garlic, minced
- 2 lbs. fresh kale or Swiss chard, stemmed and torn into large pieces
- 2 tsp. curry powder
- Freshly ground black pepper to taste

So you'll have to soak the beans overnight in enough cold water to cover by at least 2 inches. The next day drain, rinse beans well and combine in large saucepan with 4 cups water. Bring to a boil, reduce heat and simmer, covered, until beans are tender - for about 1 hour.

Meanwhile, in large, deep saucepan, heat olive oil over medium heat. Then add onion and garlic and cook, stirring often, until onion is soft - for about 5 minutes. Add greens to saucepan. Add 2 tablespoons water. Cook, tossing often, until greens are bright green - for about 3 minutes.

You can drain beans and transfer to serving dish. Then add curry powder and stir will.

Finally reheat greens and add to beans - toss to mix. Season with pepper to taste.

Nutrition Facts - Adzuki Beans

Adzuki bean - raw

Amount Per 100 grams

Calories	329

% Daily Value*	
Total Fat 0.5 g	0%
Saturated fat 0.2 g	1%
Polyunsaturated fat 0.1 g	
Monounsaturated fat 0 g	
Cholesterol 0 mg	0%
Sodium 5 mg	0%
Potassium 1,254 mg	35%
Total Carbohydrate 63 g	21%
Dietary fiber 13 g	52%
Protein 20 g	40%
Vitamin A	0%
Vitamin C	0%
Calcium	6%
Iron	27%
Vitamin D	0%
Vitamin B-6	20%
Vitamin B-12	0%
Magnesium	31%

10. Spinach Smoothie

Spinach is another power food packed with heart-healthy nutrients like potassium, folate, and magnesium — key ingredients for lowering and maintaining blood pressure levels.

Spinach is also an excellent source of vitamin K, vitamin A, vitamin C and folic acid as well as being a good source of manganese, magnesium, iron and vitamin B2. Vitamin K is important for maintaining bone health and very few vegetables are richer in Vitamin K.

Also Spinach is low in calories and high in fiber - which helps you go to the toilet.

Spinach makes a great side dish to most meals and I would also certainly recommend steaming Spinach and not boiling the goodness out of it.

Spinach Smoothie

Ingredients

- 2 cups of stemmed Spinach
- handful of grapes
- 1 x Mango
- 1 table spoon of lime juice (add more for taste)
- half a cup of Ice to thicken

Mix in blender for 2 minutes - enjoy!

Nutrition Facts - Spinach

Spinach

Amount Per 100 grams

Calories	23

% Daily Value*	
Total Fat 0.4 g	0%
Saturated fat 0.1 g	0%
Polyunsaturated fat	0.2 g
Monounsaturated fat	0 g
Cholesterol 0 mg	0%
Sodium 79 mg	3%
Potassium 558 mg	15%
Total Carbohydrate 3.6 g	1%
Dietary fiber 2.2 g	8%
Sugar 0.4 g	
Protein 2.9 g	5%
Vitamin A	187%
Vitamin C	46%
Calcium	9%
Iron	15%
Vitamin D	0%
Vitamin B-6	10%
Vitamin B-12	0%
Magnesium	19%

11. Frozen Banana Smoothie

One medium banana provides 1% of the calcium, 8% of the magnesium, and 12% of the potassium you need every day.

As we know already potassium reduces blood pressure. By relaxing the tension of arteries and veins, the blood can flow more smoothly through the body and oxygenate the various organs to increase their function.

Bananas have been linked to reducing the danger towards the kidneys from a number of different conditions. Potassium helps to regulate the fluid balance in the body, and that can help ease the strain on the kidneys, and also encouraging urination. So all in all another fantastic super food.

Frozen Banana Smoothie

Ingredients

- 2 Frozen Bananas
- 1 Apple
- 500ml of water or Almond Milk

Try peeling a few bananas - putting them in a bag and freezing them over night. Then putting them in a blender in the morning for a delicious smoothie. Add an apple and milk/almond milk/ice and extra fruit for extra flavour.

Nutrition Facts - Banana

Banana

Amount Per 100 grams

Calories	89

% Daily Value*	
Total Fat 0.3 g	0%
Saturated fat 0.1 g	0%
Polyunsaturated fat 0.1 g	
Monounsaturated fat 0 g	
Cholesterol 0 mg	0%
Sodium 1 mg	0%
Potassium 358 mg	10%
Total Carbohydrate 23 g	7%
Dietary fiber 2.6 g	10%
Sugar 12 g	
Protein 1.1 g	2%
Vitamin A	1%
Vitamin C	14%
Calcium	0%
Iron	1%
Vitamin D	0%
Vitamin B-6	20%
Vitamin B-12	0%
Magnesium	6%

One medium banana provides 1% of the calcium, 8% of the magnesium, and 12% of the potassium you need every day.

As we know already potassium reduces blood pressure. By relaxing the tension of arteries and veins, the blood can flow more smoothly through the body and oxygenate the various organs to increase their function.

Bananas have been linked to reducing the danger towards the kidneys from a number of different conditions. Potassium helps to regulate the fluid balance in the body, and that can help ease the strain on the kidneys, and also encouraging urination. So all in all another fantastic super food.

Frozen Banana Smoothie

Try peeling a few bananas - putting them in a bag and freezing them over night. Then putting them in a blender in the morning for a delicious smoothie. Add an apple and milk/almond milk/ice and extra fruit for extra flavour.

12. Kiwifruit Smoothie

Kiwifruit is delicious and just one provides 2% of the calcium, 7% of the magnesium, and 9% of the potassium you need every day.

Researchers conducted an 8 week study giving men 3 kiwi fruit a day. They found they enjoyed a drop of 10 mmHg in systolic blood pressure (top number) and 9 mmHg is diastolic blood pressure (bottom number).

At the start of the study, 65 percent were found to have normal/high-normal blood pressure, but after eight weeks, that dropped to just 33 percent.

Those figures speak for themselves. So perhaps launching into 3 kiwifruit a day is a little over the top, but having one day will reap fantastic benefits.

They also contain more vitamin C than a same-size serving of orange slices.

Kiwi Smoothie

Ingredients

- 2 kiwi fruits
- 1 apple
- 1/3 cup orange juice
- handful of ice

Slice up your kiwis and apple and put in the blender. Now throw in the rest of your ingredients in the blender. Add water to thin if too thick.

Blend for 3 minutes.

Nutrition Facts - Kiwi Fruit

Kiwi

Amount Per 100 grams

Calories 61

% Daily Value*

Total Fat 0.5 g	0%
Saturated fat 0 g	0%
Polyunsaturated fat 0.3 g	
Monounsaturated fat 0 g	
Cholesterol 0 mg	0%
Sodium 3 mg	0%

Potassium 312 mg	8%
Total Carbohydrate 15 g	5%
Dietary fiber 3 g	12%
Sugar 9 g	
Protein 1.1 g	2%
Vitamin A	1%
Vitamin C	154%
Calcium	3%
Iron	1%
Vitamin D	0%
Vitamin B-6	5%
Vitamin B-12	0%
Magnesium	4%

13. Baked Potato

Baked white potatoes are rich in both magnesium and potassium (46% of daily requirement per serving) lowers blood pressure, since potassium functions as a vasodilator.

They are full of Fiber which is also connected with scraping cholesterol out of the arteries and blood vessels, thereby increasing heart health.

Certain types of potatoes, particularly red and russet potatoes, contain high levels of flavonoid antioxidants and vitamin A, like zeaxanthin and carotenes. They can protect you against many types of cancer.

Something to consider is they should be avoided if the high blood pressure is a result of diabetes.

The Perfect Baked Potato

Firstly wash the potatoes well and then dry them - Prick several times with a fork. Get some olive oil into your hands and rub well over the potatoes. Place directly on the shelf in the oven and bake for 1¼-1½ hours, depending on the size of the potato.

Once cooked the potato should be golden-brown and crisp on the outside and give a little when pressed.

Serve split open with a healthy filling of your choice.

Nutrition Facts - Baked Potato

Potato

Amount Per 100 grams

Calories	93
% Daily Value*	
Total Fat 0.1 g	0%
Saturated fat 0 g	0%
Polyunsaturated fat 0.1 g	
Monounsaturated fat 0 g	
Cholesterol 0 mg	0%
Sodium 10 mg	0%
Potassium 535 mg	15%
Total Carbohydrate 21 g	7%
Dietary fiber 2.2 g	8%
Sugar 1.2 g	
Protein 2.5 g	5%
Vitamin A	0%
Vitamin C	16%
Calcium	1%
Iron	6%
Vitamin D	0%
Vitamin B-6	15%
Vitamin B-12	0%
Magnesium	7%

Baked white potatoes are rich in both magnesium and potassium (46% of daily requirement per serving) lowers blood pressure, since potassium functions as a vasodilator.

They are full of Fiber which is also connected with scraping cholesterol out of the arteries and blood vessels, thereby increasing heart health.

Certain types of potatoes, particularly red and russet potatoes, contain high levels of flavonoid antioxidants and vitamin A, like zeaxanthin and carotenes. They can protect you against many types of cancer.

Something to consider is they should be avoided if the high blood pressure is a result of diabetes.

The perfect Baked Potato

Firstly wash the potatoes well and then dry them - Prick several times with a fork. Get some olive oil into your hands and rub well over the potatoes. Place directly on the shelf in the oven and bake for 1¼-1½ hours, depending on the size of the potato.

Once cooked the potato should be golden-brown and crisp on the outside and give a little when pressed.

Serve split open with a healthy filling of your choice.

14. Red Bell Pepper Soup

Red peppers contain almost 300 percent of your daily vitamin C intake. That figure alone is pretty impressive!

One cup of raw red bell pepper provides 1% of the calcium, 4% of the magnesium, and 9% of the potassium you need every day.

Red peppers are one of the highest veggies in lycopene, which has been successfully tested in the prevention of many cancers including prostate and lung. The combined effects of vitamin A and C create a great antioxidant capacity, and with lycopene in the mix, the red bell pepper is a top notch superfood.

Red Pepper Soup

Ingredients

- 6 large red bell peppers, stemmed and cored, halved lengthwise, and pressed flat
- 1 tablespoon olive oil
- 4 shallots, peeled and chopped
- 1 teaspoon salt
- 1/4 teaspoon cayenne
- 1 quart fat-skimmed chicken broth
- 1 head cauliflower, cut into florets
- 1 teaspoon sugar
- Freshly ground pepper

Perfect for the winter - Preheat oven to high. Arrange bell peppers skin side up on baking sheet. Grill until skins are blackened - around 10 minutes. Then remove peppers from oven and let cool. Peel over a bowl to collect juices.

In a large pot over medium-high heat, warm olive oil. Then add shallots, salt, and cayenne and cook for 3 minutes until soft. Add Chicken broth and cauliflower. Bring to a boil, then lower heat to a simmer. Cover and cook 20 minutes. Add peppers with juices and cook, covered, until cauliflower is tender - for around 10 minutes. Purée in batches in a blender. Add pepper to taste.

Serve hot or cold and add a squeeze of lemon juice if you fancy.

Nutrition Facts - Red Bell Pepper

Amount Per 100 grams

Calories	31

% Daily Value*	
Total Fat 0.3 g	0%
Saturated fat 0 g	0%
Polyunsaturated fat 0.1 g	
Monounsaturated fat 0 g	
Cholesterol 0 mg	0%
Sodium 4 mg	0%

Potassium 211 mg	6%
Total Carbohydrate 6 g	2%
Dietary fiber 2.1 g	8%
Sugar 4.2 g	
Protein 1 g	2%
Vitamin A	62%
Vitamin C	212%
Calcium	0%
Iron	2%
Vitamin D	0%
Vitamin B-6	15%
Vitamin B-12	0%
Magnesium	3%

15. Sunflower Seeds

Sunflower seeds are also a great source of magnesium which helps reduce the severity of asthma, lower high blood pressure, and prevent migraine headaches, as well as reducing the risk of heart attack and stroke.

Sunflower seeds are a great source of vitamin E which plays an important role in the prevention of cardiovascular disease. Studies show that people who get a good amount of vitamin E are at a much lower risk of dying of a heart attack than people whose dietary intake of vitamin E isn't as good.

A handful of seeds is easy to have as a mid-morning or afternoon snack.

Breakfast

Add sunflower seeds to your breakfast - sprinkle on a table spoonful across your muesli or granola.

Nutrition Facts - Sunflower Seeds

Sunflower seeds - dried

Amount Per 100 grams

Calories	584

% Daily Value*	
Total Fat 51 g	78%
Saturated fat 4.5 g	22%
Polyunsaturated fat 23 g	
Monounsaturated fat 19 g	
Cholesterol 0 mg	0%
Sodium 9 mg	0%
Potassium 645 mg	18%
Total Carbohydrate 20 g	6%
Dietary fiber 9 g	36%
Sugar 2.6 g	
Protein 21 g	42%
Vitamin A	1%
Vitamin C	2%
Calcium	7%
Iron	28%
Vitamin D	0%
Vitamin B-6	65%
Vitamin B-12	0%
Magnesium	81%

16. Milk - for a great night's sleep

Drinking low-fat milk will provide you with calcium and vitamin D — the two nutrients work as a team to help reduce blood pressure by 3 to 10 percent.

One cup of milk has half of the recommended daily allowance of B12. However something to bear in mind is that milk also has lactose, so it can cause gastrointestinal or digestive problems for people who have a deficiency of the lactase enzyme. This typically causes bloating - so avoid if this doesn't get on with you.

Hot Milk before Bed

Drinking a glass of warm milk before bed will help you to sleep better. Dairy products are rich in the amino acid tryptophan, which helps in the production of the sleep inducing brain chemicals, serotonin and melatonin. Try it!

Nutrition Facts - Milk

Milk - 1% fat

Amount Per 100 grams

Calories	42

% Daily Value*

Total Fat 1 g	1%
Saturated fat 0.6 g	3%
Polyunsaturated fat 0 g	
Monounsaturated fat 0.3 g	
Cholesterol 5 mg	1%
Sodium 44 mg	1%
Potassium 150 mg	4%
Total Carbohydrate 5 g	1%
Dietary fiber 0 g	0%
Sugar 5 g	
Protein 3.4 g	6%
Vitamin A	0%
Vitamin C	0%
Calcium	12%
Iron	0%
Vitamin D	0%
Vitamin B-6	0%
Vitamin B-12	8%
Magnesium	2%

17. Soybean Salad

Soybeans are another excellent source of potassium and magnesium - great for crushing that high blood pressure down.

Also clinical trials found that 20 g to 61 g of soy protein a day can significantly reduce total blood cholesterol levels, LDL (bad) cholesterol levels and triglycerides. The results also showed that soy protein supplementation slightly increased HDL (good) cholesterol levels. Again positive news for a healthy cardiovascular system.

Before washing dried soybeans, spread them out on a dark colored plate or cooking surface to check for and remove small stones, debris or damaged beans. After this process, place the beans in a strainer and rinse them thoroughly under cool running water.

Soybean Salad

Ingredients

- 16 oz Can of Black soybeans, drained and rinsed
- 1 cup Drained canned or cooked corn kernels
- 1 cup Sliced celery
- 1/2 cup Diced sweet red peppers and green peppers
- 1/4 cup Sliced green onions and ripe olive

- 1/4 cup Soybean oil (vegetable oil) and white wine vinegar
- 1/2 teaspoon Chili powder

This is a very easy and quick dish - one of my favorites. Combine drained soybeans, corn, celery, sweet peppers, green onions, olives and hot peppers in a large bowl; toss to mix. Combine remaining ingredients in a small bowl and blend all ingredients. Add some freshly ground pepper to taste. Pour dressing over soybean mixture and marinate at least 1 hour. Then serve cold - perfect!

Nutrition Facts - Soybeans

Soybeans - raw

Amount Per 100 grams

Calories	446

% Daily Value*	
Total Fat 20 g	30%
Saturated fat 2.9 g	14%
Polyunsaturated fat 11 g	
Monounsaturated fat 4.4 g	
Cholesterol 0 mg	0%
Sodium 2 mg	0%
Potassium 1,797 mg	51%
Total Carbohydrate 30 g	10%
Dietary fiber 9 g	36%
Sugar 7 g	

Protein 36 g	72%
Vitamin A	0%
Vitamin C	10%
Calcium	27%
Iron	87%
Vitamin D	0%
Vitamin B-6	20%
Vitamin B-12	0%
Magnesium	70%

18. Talipa Tacos

Just four ounces of Tilapia provides 8% of the magnesium and 8% of the potassium you need every day.

Tilapia is extremely low in environmental toxins like mercury and PCBs (polychlorinated biphenyls), and it is considered a sustainable, environmentally friendly choice.

In the US Tilapia is grown in closed-system fish farms on plant-based diets. This doesn't threaten stocks of wild fish according to the nonprofit Food & Water Watch.

Tilapia Tacos With Cucumber

Ingredients

- 1 tablespoon olive oil, plus more for the grill
- 4 6-ounce tilapia, halibut, or black bass fillets
- 1 teaspoon ground coriander
- kosher salt and black pepper
- 6 radishes, sliced
- 1 cucumber, halved and sliced
- 2 tablespoons fresh lime juice, plus lime wedges for serving
- 8 corn tortillas, warmed
- 1 cup fresh cilantro leaves
- 1/4 cup sour cream

So let's heat grill to high and add oil grill. Then season the fish with the coriander, adding the ½ teaspoon salt, and the ¼ teaspoon pepper and grill until cooked through, 1 to 2 minutes per side.

Use a medium bowl, toss the radishes and cucumber with the lime juice, oil, and ¼ teaspoon each salt and pepper.

Serve the fish in the tortillas with the cucumber relish, cilantro, sour cream, and lime wedges and enjoy!

Nutrition Facts - Talipa

Tilapia - cooked

Amount Per 100 grams

Calories	129

% Daily Value*	
Total Fat 2.6 g	4%
Saturated fat 0.9 g	4%
Polyunsaturated fat 0.6 g	
Monounsaturated fat 1 g	
Cholesterol 57 mg	19%
Sodium 56 mg	2%
Potassium 380 mg	10%
Total Carbohydrate 0 g	0%
Dietary fiber 0 g	0%
Sugar 0 g	
Protein 26 g	52%
Vitamin A	0%
Vitamin C	0%
Calcium	1%
Iron	3%

Vitamin D	37%
Vitamin B-6	5%
Vitamin B-12	31%
Magnesium	8%

19. Sweet Potato Mash

One of my favorite carbohydrate sources is sweet potato. A medium sweet potato with the skin provides 4% of the calcium, 8% of the magnesium (7% without the skin), and 15% of the potassium (10% without the skin) you need every day.

Sweet potatoes are rich in beta-carotene which can help ward off free radicals that damage cells through oxidation. Free radicals speed up aging and make you vulnerable against chronic diseases. This antioxidant can help support your immune system, as well as lower your risk of heart disease and cancer.

These vegetables are also great sources of vitamins C and B5, copper, dietary fiber, niacin, potassium, and iron

Sweet Potato Mash

Ingredients

- 500g carrots, chopped
- 500g sweet potatoes, chopped
- 3 garlic cloves, bashed
- 1 tsp cumin seeds, toasted
- 25g butter

One of my favs - Add the carrots, sweet potatoes and garlic in a large pan of salted water, bring to the boil, then cook for 12 mins. Then add cumin seeds, butter and seasoning. Roughly mash it all together - it doesn't have to be perfect. Then serve.

Nutrition Facts - Sweet Potato

Amount Per 100 grams

Calories	86

% Daily Value*	
Total Fat 0 g	0%
Saturated fat 0 g	0%
Polyunsaturated fat 0 g	
Monounsaturated fat 0 g	
Cholesterol 0 mg	0%
Sodium 55 mg	2%
Potassium 337 mg	9%
Total Carbohydrate 20 g	6%
Dietary fiber 3 g	12%
Sugar 4.2 g	
Protein 1.6 g	3%
Vitamin A	283%
Vitamin C	4%
Calcium	3%
Iron	3%
Vitamin D	0%
Vitamin B-6	10%
Vitamin B-12	0%
Magnesium	6%

20. Quinoa and Lentil Salad

Quinoa is a high-protein whole grain contains a variety of health-protecting phytonutrients along with an impressive amount of magnesium. Quinoa is gluten free, making it a great option if you're gluten intolerant or have celiac disease.

A half-cup of cooked Quinoa provides 1.5% of the calcium, 15% of the magnesium, and 4.5% of the potassium you need every day. Magnesium helps to relax blood vessels and thereby to alleviate migraines.

Quinoa contains almost twice as much fiber as most other grains. All in all this is a super food that you can't go wrong with and easy to cook.

Quinoa Salad

Ingredients

- 200g Quinoa
- 1 tsp olive oil
- 1 shallot or ½ onion, finely chopped
- 2 tbsp tarragon, roughly chopped
- 14oz 400g can Puy or green lentils rinsed and drained
- ¼ cucumber, lightly peeled and diced

- 100g feta cheese, crumbled
- 6 spring onions, thinly sliced
- zest and juice 1 orange
- 1 tbsp red or white wine vinegar

This is a super tasty meal. Cook the quinoa in a large pan of boiling water for 10-15 mins until soft, drain well, then set aside to cool.

Meanwhile, heat the oil in a small pan, and then cook the shallot or onion for a few minutes until softened. Add the tarragon, stir well, then remove from the heat.

Finally stir the softened shallot and tarragon into the cooled quinoa along with the lentils, cucumber, feta, spring onions, orange zest and juice and vinegar. Mix well together and chill until ready to serve - enjoy!

Nutrition Facts - Quinoa

Quinoa - uncooked

Amount Per 100 grams

Calories	368

% Daily Value*	
Total Fat 6 g	9%
Saturated fat 0.7 g	3%
Polyunsaturated fat 3.3 g	

Monounsaturated fat 1.6 g	
Cholesterol 0 mg	0%
Sodium 5 mg	0%
Potassium 563 mg	16%
Total Carbohydrate 64 g	21%
Dietary fiber 7 g	28%
Protein 14 g	28%
Vitamin A	0%
Vitamin C	0%
Calcium	4%
Iron	25%
Vitamin D	0%
Vitamin B-6	25%
Vitamin B-12	0%
Magnesium	49%

21. Avocado Smoothie

One-half of an avocado provides 1% of the calcium, 5% of the magnesium, and 10% of the potassium you need every day. This is very high potassium level - higher than Bananas - which should support healthy blood pressure levels. Avocados are high in monounsaturated oleic acid - a "heart healthy" fatty acid.

Avocados also contain a huge amount of Fiber and heart-healthy monounsaturated fats and health-promoting carotenoids.

Avocados are great to add to main meals including chicken dishes or salads.

Avocado Smoothie

Ingredients

- 1 frozen banana (the riper the sweeter)
- ½ a California Avocado
- ½ cup almond milk
- A touch of honey or agave

Blend together for a kickstart to the day - the perfect breakfast on the go.

Nutrition Facts - Avocado

Amount Per 100 grams

Calories	160
% Daily Value*	
Total Fat 15 g	23%
Saturated fat 2.1 g	10%
Polyunsaturated fat 1.8 g	
Monounsaturated fat 10 g	
Cholesterol 0 mg	0%
Sodium 7 mg	0%
Potassium 485 mg	13%
Total Carbohydrate 9 g	3%
Dietary fiber 7 g	28%
Sugar 0.7 g	
Protein 2 g	4%
Vitamin A	2%
Vitamin C	16%
Calcium	1%
Iron	3%
Vitamin D	0%
Vitamin B-6	15%
Vitamin B-12	0%
Magnesium	7%

22. Rounding off...

So well done for making it to the end. I truly hope that you follow at least some of the ideas here as they can make a tremendous difference to not only reducing your blood pressure but your overall health.

The recipes I've included are ideas, the most important thing are that these foods contain nutrients that can help lower your blood pressure and you can be as creative as you want.

Start with small changes and then build up to healthy eating 5 out of 7 days up to 6 out of 7. I would recommend having a 'relaxed' day, this is when you can eat what you want. Otherwise you'll feel deprived and the whole thing becomes a chore. It isn't. This is for you. But YOU must want to change.

Here are a number of other things that will greatly reduce your high blood pressure:

- Take up some light Exercise daily
- Limit the alcohol in your diet
- Quit smoking (if you do)
- Cut back on Caffeine
- Try to manage your stress. This is a lot easier said than done when you have a full time job and responsibilities. However consider going for a walk

at lunch, or before dinner. Try to cut off your work time so you can relax in the evening. Small things help.

Please review this book as it helps me continue my work into lowering blood pressure and other remedies to help us deal with problems safely and naturally.

Finally good luck with lowering your blood pressure, I know it will be worth it.

--M

Printed in Great Britain
by Amazon